# *FIT AFTER FORTY*

## *– My Journey:*

## *Part One*

# DEDICATION

To my wife. She always did nag me about completing one work at least. There you go Missy!


Preferred author at writimg.com, 'dragon online'. You read my first draft and gave me the sort of commendation that left me no room to back off. Thanks, lots.


That should do it, I think.

*"Tis in ourselves that we are thus or thus. Our bodies are our gardens to the which our wills are gardeners."*

*-  William Shakespeare, Othello*

# INTRODUCTION

How to do this. What is this?

Had to take a peek at a list of types of published work to get a shady fix on this one.

A memoir of sorts? Perhaps. But, hopefully, one that will prove anecdotal yet instructive, in essence. Nomenclatural procedures of published work in the literary parlance not of particular interest so, how about you call it whatever you will. You *should* probably read on a bit if you insist on categorization though. Otherwise, just follow along on this journey of mine. And yes, I do promise zero predictability.

You see, it's my run at the dreaded middle ages – age forty-five in my case - and I came upon a certain, not fleeting, drive. A surge of will, if you will. I had an unshakeable drive to accomplish something (hardly an occurrence for me), and it had everything to do with my body.

The *journey* begins.

I remember back in the day, in chemistry class. The word 'catalyst' intrigued me somewhat. Can't say why specifically. The thought it conveyed perhaps. I imagined very violent chemical reactions triggered by drops of some mild liquid. I found it curious how such profound reactions could be sparked off by an unassuming action. What triggered, catalyzed the series of events in this journey of mine was just as unassuming. The results though? Well, you'll see.

Had an itch in my groin. It was one of those itches that came on suddenly and required immediate action. So, I acted. I realized however, that I had grown what looked and felt like my own personal patch of the amazon right there in my groin. Had to sift through rough 'foliage' to get to that itch.

I let out a sigh. It amused me how neglectful I had been of my 'area'. So, I took out a shaving stick and did the thing. Well, I tried to. Problem was, I couldn't see the damned 'forest'. Bad old mid-ages belly fat was in the way! Shouldn't have been shocked, but I was. Took years to get to that point, but it only took that one moment to fully realize how much of my abdominals had been copiously covered by fat. I could hardly even see my genitals without some tedious tummy tucking-in, and only some of it at that. Shaving? That was practically impossible if I had to rely on mere line of sight without using a mirror. This all hit me quite hard.

How? When did this happen??!!

It was there all along, years in the making. I just never really noticed; until that moment. The micro-events of that morning in the bathroom constituted the 'catalyst' for me. A damned good one too, except it wasn't the only one. It was clear *what* I had to do. Simple really. Except, 'simple' didn't quite cut it. *Knowing* what to do about something and actually *doing* it, is no package deal. Get in shape, or back in it (I do have some shady memory of a time I was kind of fit), was what I had to do. First though, I had to see to a doctor's appointment in a couple hours.

So, the doctor tells me the recent, frequent headaches I'd been having were because I was hypertensive and apparently didn't even know it. Second shock of the day. Rather odd I'd have two 'epic', life-altering events occur in one 24-hour period. Here was life throwing me 2 rotten apples in one day. How utterly cruel.

I always (ridiculously) prided myself on possessing one of those 'physiological constitutions' that resisted such conditions as hypertension, and most other conditions for that matter. I figured since I had only ever known asthma (and later, chronic bronchitis), as personal ailments, I was perhaps immune to other conditions. As a kid, my asthma was some invisible 'caped wonder' protecting me from any and all other illnesses. I only had to suffer the 'inconvenience' of the occasional trip to the ER to treat severe attacks as 'appeasement'. Laughable really, if not just plain quixotic, especially when you considered the fact that I held this ludicrous delusion for most of my adult life. *Even as I studied science pretty much all my schooling years.* My asthma didn't lose its 'caped hero' status a few years ago when I first battled chronic bronchitis, but it diminished somewhat. My discovery of having hypertension however, completely vaporized this life-long hero friend and protector. Time to wake up and smell the repugnant roses of a world full of wretched ailments.

Moving on.

So, my composite catalyst, although comprising a couple or more micro-elements not worth mentioning, was complete. I really, really had to get fit again. And body aesthetics was now not even a serious consideration. My overall health was at stake here. The doctor listed lifestyle changes I had to make. All of which, by training, I already knew – even touted. Never did practice what I preached. I knew the science. Taught it at some euphoric point in my life even. It was time to start my journey to fitness and I was concretely determined. Nothing whimsical here (and I *have* been known to be more than a little capricious), and perhaps one of the very few times in my life I would be summoning a resource of will I knew I had but hardly (I mean really hardly) ever used. This was it then.

The next three months would be the hardest, sexiest, most exhilarating of my life. Not sure why I included 'sexiest' in the foregoing, but it felt right to be there. So, it stays. Will probably get around to explaining why my fingers went to those particular letters while typing that line; at some point anyway (wide grin).

So, what precipitated my quest for fitness after forty? Think I got that out of the way.

To be sure, much of what comes next is my overall experience using proven techniques based on sound science (and not a little grit), towards losing unhealthy fat and gaining useful, lean muscle in all the right places. I never quite followed a strict, recommended regimen, but developed my very own routine based on my knowledge of how the body works, at rest and in movement; as well as gleaning useful 'stuff' from effortful research done by others.

It is my hope that, if you're male and over forty, grappling with a waistline that does very little for your self-esteem; looking to gain a measure of physical fitness that will drive your good-health index upward; and would really, really like to do something the hell about it, you will find this an informative and beneficial read. This is no fitness manual, although perhaps I actually am qualified to create one. This is the journey of a man like you, with real concerns and agitations about his overall health and wellbeing. Being fit over forty does more than you could possibly fathom for your state of mind, your physical capacity (and yes this does include, but is not limited to, your prowess between the sheets) to carry out daily tasks, and your overall sense of 'being'. You may find your interactions with others also get a make-over.

This is my story, as a human being above all else, summoning the will (and maintaining it) to make worthwhile changes. It wasn't a walk in the park as you will see, but the benefits of the sail *were* worth the turbulence. The shore? Exquisite!

My original script next went like, "Don't expect a content list." Well, that was until my publisher insisted on a content table. So, I've provided one. Still, don't expect it to point you in any predictable direction - for the most part. Won't be much of an adventure if it did, would it? Really would be nice if you came on this trip with me; you might find it quite the enlightening one. So why not? Do come along now.

Here we go. The quest itself.

Ever heard the term, 'intermittent fasting'?

Well, me neither. At least not before my quest began. I did, however, find the theory sound. Put simply, you deprive yourself of food (this includes beverages with significant caloric content) for a predetermined number of hours daily, restricting your eating period to a finite amount of time. Now, there are several ways to do this. However, *I* chose to go the 16/8 route. This meant that I would go without food 16 hours during a 24-hour (full day) period, limiting food intake to the remaining 8 hours. You can, however take water, coffee (no milk or sugar), or some other liquid with very little or no caloric content.

### *The Theory*

Did I mention I weighed 85kg by the time my journey began? Pretty sure I did not. For a height of 5'8", it meant I was sufficiently overweight to flirt with the obesity borderline. The brooding, dark figure with the mad grin (I often visualized) – obesity – beckoned from the other side. I was probably, no - I was in fact inexorably moving towards the insane lure of that figure when the catalyst happened.

Food is what keeps you alive. Fact. Unfortunately, it is one thing that could also kill you. Too much of it, and for too long.

I knew I had to rethink my eating routine. Enter, Intermittent Fasting.

Again, this isn't a scientific paper so I'm going to make this as understandable as possible, without sacrificing essential details of course; hopefully.

So, the theory here is quite simple. When the human body is deprived of food for more than 12 hours, a number of interesting things begin to happen. For one, the body starts to turn to fat stores to provide needed energy to do work. Now, research is ongoing to fully establish the intricate processes here, but several facts have been determined; like the one I enunciated a few lines up. For someone intending to whittle down those fatty deposits then, intermittent fasting was one method I found to be expedient as I journeyed.

The key is to deny the body food for between 12 to 18 hours (max) if you're doing the 16/8 routine. You've got to keep at it though. The 16/8 method is really quite as easy as simply skipping breakfast and restricting lunch and dinner to a 6-8-hour period. Tough the first few days if you previously took breakfast quite seriously, but persistence is gold here. However, as long as the fasting period lasts for the recommended period, you can do breakfast (if you're a stickler) while adjusting your other meals to fit in with the program. For instance, you could have your treasured 'brekkie' and lunch within a 6-8-hour window and skip dinner. Same deal, different routes. How does this work exactly? Here it comes.

Imagine your regular power generator. You got a tank full of fuel, yes? But regular power is out, and no way of telling when that'll return. So, you shore up. Now, the generator's tank runs dry so you go fetch your store of fuel. Well, you hoped you wouldn't have to do this, but prepared for it nonetheless.

The body, like that generator uses the fuel in its go-to tank to provide energy. In this case the tank of fuel is its store of glycogen. Glycogen are tiny little cells (or organic containers) that hold sugar. The body burns the sugar (or glucose) as fuel to produce energy for work. When the body runs out of its go-to fuel, it turns to its reserve store – fat cells. Fat cells contain stored energy the body can utilize to keep running. Here, the brain mobilizes some key hormones (hormones are 'messenger' substances the brain recruits to accomplish specific tasks in different areas of the body). The Human Growth Hormone (HGH) is one such messenger hormone. These hormones then act upon the fat stores causing the fat cells to break down to simpler forms (glucose) the body can use as a ready fuel source.

Now, in the case of your power generator above, the fuel stores are a backup and you really would rather not use them. In this case however, you so, so, want the body to go get that fat store and break it, break it, break it down. Intermittent fasting is our way of telling the brain you don't need those stores of fat and, to burn them. But the brain sure won't listen unless you compel it to. When you fast for the recommended period, you force your brain to resort to its programmed response – go get that fat store. And you get to grin at the accomplishment. Well, at least I did.

I mentioned somewhere above (you got to go a bit farther up I reckon) there are variations to this intermittent fasting. One other method involves whole 24-hour periods of fasting (a day or two a week) while you eat (hopefully not gorge) the rest of the weekdays. You can look up the other methods to find what best suits you.

I should mention: the 16/8 method does not necessarily require it be done every single day. You could start with 2 or more days of the week and get comfy first. Then, ramp things up. The other methods also lend pretty well to flexible plans.

So, what did *I* do in more detail? This *Is* my journey after all.

## *My Intermittent Fasting Journey*

Right off the bat, I fasted a straight 18 hours. Drank a cup or two of coffee during though. Totally permitted. Oh, and yes, apple cyder vinegar. That 'couple' did a backflip on my appetite. The point really. Studies have indeed shown coffee and cyder to be appetite suppressants. Research also indicates (although not definitive) that coffee may play a role in the body's fat burning processes, even while you're at rest. You don't want to overdo the coffee though, especially if you're hypertensive as I am. Also, you *might* want to take them (coffee and cyder) independently of each other – you just know I couldn't resist combining, and the results were sublimely unpleasant (yuck!).

So, armed with my arsenal of coffee and apple cyder vinegar, my intermittent fasting journey kicked off.

Now, I chose to keep my 'eating window' between 12noon and 6pm. Worked just fine for me. I was also careful not to binge-eat during the period. That sort of defeats the purpose doesn't it?

What to eat? That is entirely up to you. However, a few tips might be in order, for best results. One would be that you do less carbs and more protein. Protein is that food class your muscles absolutely need to strengthen and grow. I was looking to lose the fat and gain 'lean body mass'. Put simply, lean body mass = total body weight – fat mass. 'Muscle mass' refers quite strictly to your muscular composition (muscles alone). So, as a targeted result, I aimed to retain and perhaps increase my 'muscle mass' while getting rid of undesirable fat.

Keep in mind: consuming large portions of carbs will provide your body with an immediate source of energy, yes, but when the body has used what it needs, it converts the rest into fat, ultimately. You don't want that. Be moderate with your carbs intake and do more protein instead. The protein won't swell your fat deposits but will do wonders for your muscle mass, with the additional benefit of making you feel fuller without needing to gorge yourself. You follow?

Eggs are a fine source of protein. Lean meat like poultry and fish are also excellent sources.

Another tip: You don't want to overlook them vegetables. They do more than add textural variations and color to your food. They're actually good for you.

So, more protein and veggies. Less carbs. Winning formula any day.

For me, a typical intermittent-fasting-day would begin with a cup of coffee and, sometime later, a short glass of apple cyder vinegar-water combo. And then at noon, do some veggie-protein-carb cocktail, keeping the proportions as recommended above. It was quite the creative journey for me in many ways. I constantly had to concoct some variant form of the 'cocktail' to sustain my interest, not to mention determination to keep at it. The Food Network channel became my emergency buddy as I found a plethora of ideas and inspiration there to keep me sufficiently committed to the new eating plan.

"What the hell is that!?", my wife exclaimed one day she chanced upon one of my cocktail, mad-scientist creations. To be fair, I didn't quite get it myself. It *was* quite hideous. It was an incongruous assembly of ingredients that had no business being on the same plate (better in their respective compartments in the pantry yes, but certainly not combined that way using *oh* precious heat). However, although it was culinary grotesquery on display, the taste was a different matter entirely. No point detailing what my cocktail contained. *Needless to offend culinary sensibilities here, although I am tempted to for the sadistic fun of it*. My point is, play around with your food (pun intended), using healthy choices for ingredients of course. Why stick to stereotypes when you can make eating healthy a challenge each time you make your own food. A gross looking plate of food containing healthy ingredients, in the most beneficial proportions, won't give you points on 'Chopped', but will score you valuable points when a healthy body is your prize.

The intermittent fasting routine, since limiting my eating window to between 12 and 6pm meant that I always had an early dinner. That is generally a good habit. Whenever I felt hungry after dinner, I would do another cup of coffee or more of that sordid cyder-water mixture (don't have to like what helps you). Worked spectacularly.

In time, my body got used to the whole routine. Sweet. It meant, among other things, I had far fewer dreams of sitting in the middle of a fete-worthy spread of the tastiest looking food and, suddenly, having it all snatched away by unseen, wicked hands. Those were the worst, at first. The hateful dreams stopped, eventually. Got to hand it to this body of ours. It does get the 'message' soon enough. So, without meaning to flog the issue, you really have to keep at this to reap the rewards. Oh, you're going to slip up. We're not robots with flawless programming. When you pick up right after and continue right on, those slip-ups only get fewer till they disappear altogether.

I had zero slip-ups.

But, for me it was a question of far greater weight than the initial goal. I had something to prove. I never quite followed anything of importance to its desired end-point. This was my chance - one chance - to prove to yours truly ('moi') I could see something of value to its desired conclusion. No slip-ups didn't mean it was some cakewalk, however. And I'm not here referring to my intermittent fasting journey alone. The whole shebang. As you will see (hopefully in a short while), my entire journey was quite the robust one.

Come with me then....as, the *Journey* continues.

You see, I was hoping for the shortcut in my journey. Remember when I said I absolutely needed to see this 'thing' through? So…I was convinced I could do it in the shortest amount of time. Trepidation at falling back to my routine of *not* seeing things through, I sought to minimize the risk (at least). In my pre-journey research, I came upon good old *Tabata.* Don't know why, but 'Tabata' always did conjure up 'Shakespearish' images in my mind. Still does. Perhaps, the literary savants can find some connection. But that's irrelevant, forgive me. Tabata, however, is a real person's name. Turns out a Japanese fellow bearing the name came up with a brilliant exercise routine (oh yes, were going down and dirty into the nitty gritty of this journey – the dreaded workouts), and it was named after him.

Before I elucidate the Tabata a bit more, a little of the 'why exercise' might just be in order.

Whether you believe the human body was designed and subsequently created by some supremely intelligent being (or beings for that matter) or, that it had to evolve over the millennia to its current state of perplexing complexity, is by no means a contention here. The truth however isn't lost in such philosophical debates (never did like debates much). The truth is: the human body is amazing in complexity as it functions, as much in everyday routine activity, as it does in more refined, deliberate ones. Picking up a pencil, and performing complex Judo moves both require extraordinary musculo-skeletal coordination, for instance (not to mention the neural activity involved). Here's the thing though, as much as I would absolutely love to dive right into this incredibly complex and amazing topic of the mechanisms of movement, I cannot deviate too far from my aim of taking you on this ride of mine. Although I hope to teach what life lessons I can here, I really don't want to do too much of the 'science stuff'. So, how about we move this along, making our experience as much fun as possible while learning a thing or two. Deal?

So, here's one reason why exercise is good for you.

When I taught some undergrads back in the day (that 'euphoric' period in my life I mentioned near the beginning), I really loved to use illustrations to make things a little easier to grasp. I long since left that activity of teaching, but the penchant for using illustrations to help illuminate, lives on!

Here's one.

Think of a very complex machine. Now, this 'super' machine has moving parts that work to enable it perform at optimal levels. Now get this: this particular machine's overall efficiency, improves with the constant use of those moving parts. To be sure, the machine will still function if the moving parts are utilized less (or even not at all). However, the chances the machine will break down in that scenario increase significantly. This machine wasn't made to break down after a short spell of use. So, for best results, the machine simply must utilize those moving parts as consistently as possible. And the fact that the machine doesn't just *stay* efficient at a level degree – but gets increasingly so with the use of those moving parts makes it even more intriguing and impressive. You may be hard-pressed to find such a man-made machine. It may exist though. I simply don't know of one. Three words: wear and tear.

The human body though. Now, that's one heck of a machine. Our bodies actually become *more* efficient as we *move* more.

Our world has become so much more automated that the simplest tasks are now assigned to machines or pieces of equipment that simply – do the job for us. 'We need to move more'. Those five words seem simplistic and cliche. Yet, how much do our bodies move each day? How much is enough? If you're obese or overweight, clearly not enough. Can't get more compendious than that. Fact, theory, research, all form part of a prodigious human endeavor to try to make us move more and, to show how so much benefit results.

So, one reason exercises are good for you? Exercises provide a structured way to move that body of yours in the most productive manner, improving overall system efficiency. Yes, your body functions better as you move more through exercise. So, so, neat.


Tabata…finally.

So, it came to me eventually. Remembered why the name Tabata was reminiscent of some work the immortal Shakespeare did at some point. Wasn't Shakespeare though. I must have made that connection subliminally. The literary work part anyway. My bad. At least now the literary savants I put to task earlier need not bother (if they were actually going to).

Stephen King it was. His wife specifically, Tabitha King – bingo! King happens to be a favorite writer of mine. Just so turns out he gives his Missy a big, fat load of credit every book he writes (those I've read, to be sure). My Missy should probably get the same treatment in accolade whenever this gets published. Hopefully. *"Hope is a good thing, maybe the best of things" (Andy, Shawshank Redemption)*. Her reaction though....

So, what is this Tabata workout routine, eponymous of the Japanese fitness expert who created it?

Nitty-gritty time.

Now, a central idea of any physical workout routine is to improve the body's capacity to do physical work by strengthening the various systems that coordinate to make this happen. Key systems in this regard are the muscular, cardiovascular and respiratory. Although, others like the immune and neurological systems are also positively influenced by exercise, I'll be focusing on the previous three above. Note that I will be using 'physical workout' (or just plain 'workout) and 'exercise' interchangeably in this interaction as they both roughly refer to the same activity – structured movement regimens that are pre-planned and designed to produce desired physical capacity enhancement results. So, when you do 10 pushups for instance, you're performing a pre-planned, structured physical activity designed to build your arms, core (these are mostly the muscles of the abdominal area, lower back, pelvic area and hips), and chest muscles – or, you **workout/exercise**. Climbing a winding flight of stairs as an opposing instance, however, simply means you're engaging in physical activity. Moving on.

The muscular, cardiovascular and respiratory systems simply refer to your muscles, heart with attendant blood vessels, and your lungs. Science and fancy nomenclature are best buds. Always have been. No matter. *I* fancy breaking them down.

Here it is. *Did I say I wasn't going to get into the mechanisms of movement? Oh shucks.*

When you exercise, your muscles, heart, and lungs concertedly kick into overdrive to ensure that your body can handle the increased work. As simplistic as that looked to read, the mechanisms here are far more complex, but fear not, complex can get a whole lot less so if 'dissolved' a bit. First off, to do any physical activity, your body has to convert sources of energy into the energy itself to do the work; much like that generator I illustrated earlier burns the fuel in its store tank to produce the electrical energy we utilize. The sugars and carbohydrates we consume, provide those go-to sources of energy. When athletes (amateur and professional alike) train, that heart/lungs/muscles trio above works to enable the body accomplish the tasks involved in such training. But how? It gets interesting here. To understand Tabata, you need to have some basic information. Do follow me.

Our muscles, and connected joints, accomplish the activity of movement – at any level. For them to do so however, they need to transform glucose (sugar, simply) in their cells, in the presence of oxygen, to produce the energy required for them to do so. However, such a 'transformation' isn't a one-off thing. Any level or intensity of physical activity would require that the muscles receive a steady supply of fuel (glucose and oxygen) to do the work. How do these muscles hard at work get what they need? The heart and lungs step in. The heart for one, pumps out blood through connected vessels (your arteries) containing those two essential elements above needed for successful energy synthesis (or production). The muscles then happily receive the essential supplies and continue to work. How did the oxygen get into the blood though? Yes, you nailed it! Your lungs. When you work out, you certainly realize that your breathing becomes more insistent, a whole lot more intense. That's because your muscles need more oxygen to function optimally when engaged in more intense work than the regular, average tasks. So, your lungs which receive, contain, and supply the vital oxygen breathed in, work tirelessly to provide those active muscles their oxygen requirements. Here, the heart sends blood directly to the lungs to receive fresh oxygen for onward delivery to the working muscles. These microprocesses happen in microseconds producing 'macro-results'. Now, each individual microprocess of oxygen and glucose delivery to the muscle cells is actually a cycle. The muscle cells don't merely receive needed fuel, but also jettison waste products, this time into 'veins' which chiefly return blood with wastes back to the heart for distribution to those organs tasked with waste processing and ejection. Think of your generator again. Fuel burning creates carbon monoxide (an undesirable waste), and spews this out through exhaust pipes (the body actually did it first....yayyy!). In this regard, the lungs play a dual role. They recycle the gases involved in physical activity (as in life itself), by receiving the waste carbon dioxide ejected by the muscles after oxygen-to-energy synthesis; you then breathe it all out, and mostly only the florae are happier for it.

So, anytime you think of physical activity, whether you're exercising or you're just being human doing those mundane daily tasks that require some level of movement, I hope you can more fully appreciate the intricate processes involved. That trio - the heart, lungs and muscles - gets the job done.

Regarding how Tabata ties into all of this? Comes next.

There are probably as many variations of exercise routines as there are those who study them. In most cases, the end does justify the means. In other words, what routine you chose to implement will likely depend on what you're aiming to achieve. So, if you want to get 'buff' like Arnold the 'Schwarz' or his buddy Stallone (in their hay days anyway), you might want to focus on strength training routines. If running the next paying-marathon is your fancy, then endurance training is your 'boulevard'. Fancy Usain Bolt and his enviable speed? Then exercises that condition you to produce high energy bursts for short periods will suffice. Of course, the distinctions above aren't so strict, but they do require that each training goal adopt routines that will produce the best results, as desired.

If you're just looking to go on *my* kind of journey however, a bit of combo activity may be required.

So basically, Tabata is one form of a group of 'high intensity, short duration' exercise routines that max you out while you perform them. High-intensity interval training (HIIT) is another way of naming this group. You may find other terms like 'high-intensity intermittent exercise (HIIE) and 'sprint interval training' (SIT) if you take the leap from here to do a bit more research online. They all pretty much refer to the same thing (again with the fancy nomenclature... shucks). The crux though, is that while you perform these routines, to the point of exhaustion (no joke here), they mostly last for short periods with even shorter moments of rest. The whole idea? Follow me now.

When you go jogging for a couple or more kilometers, as an example, you're doing a 'steady-state' workout. This basically means that you're performing that physical activity at a rate your heart and lungs can sustain for that period without serious fatigue to the muscles. Remember when we touched on working muscles requiring oxygen and glucose to perform? I also indicated the fact that a by-product of muscular activity is carbon dioxide ($CO_2$) exhaled (rather diligently) by the lungs. When this cycle is performed in a state of steady oxygen supply (as with the jogging example above), this 'steady state' exercise can be performed for a considerable period of time (think marathon runners). When you do light jogging, you may observe that all along the way, you are able to breathe in and out at a fairly consistent rate. This steady supply of oxygen to the working muscles (alongside the glucose) provides the endurance needed to continue in that steady state of work for a substantial period. This type of exercise is referred to as 'aerobic' (with oxygen).

It's a whole different scenario however, when you get to perform 'high intensity' workouts. Imagine doing a sprint, a 50-meter, all-out, sweat-drenching, unforgiving sprint your life actually depended on. Well, you may have had to do this one time or another, whether for play or actual 'fight or flight' adrenal gland release response – the mechanisms are the same. You don't get the luxury of breathing in and out at a 'relaxed', steady state. Fact is, you do that 'short', very intense activity, without any fair amount of breathing. Here, we refer to anaerobic exercise (without oxygen). So, how do your muscles get the work done in the absence of adequate oxygen? Simply, it uses the available stores of glucose and 'glycogen' (glycogen is a bit more complex form of glucose stored in the liver and broken down to base level glucose for energy synthesis). Now, because it does so in the absence of oxygen, you get a by-product called 'Lactic Acid' which builds up in the muscles faster than it can be cycled off. This build-up inhibits muscle performance, hence the fatigue felt while doing intense workouts, requiring a 'ceasefire' when unbearable. But, while high intensity exercise bouts are inherently short bursts, they do pack a serious punch (you get to understand this 'serious punch' a bit more later). And, while you perform a typical HIIT (high intensity interval training) routine, there are short periods of rest interspersing. So, you have a short period of heart-bursting exercise bout followed by an even shorter period of rest, and the cycle reiterated.

Now a typical Tabata. A typical Tabata cycle will include 20-second bouts of high intensity exercises that nearly max you out (or even do so), followed by a 10 second 'recoup' period. Now, you repeat this cycle (seamlessly) eight times, to complete one full Tabata. In all, you spend 4 minutes. A blast (If by blast you can conjure up the sensation of actually being blasted by a grenade magnitude force, then yeah)!

As an example. You spot-sprint (or sprinting on the spot: imagine you're running the 50-meter dash standing in one spot, then actually do it) for 20 seconds followed by a 10 second 'catch-your-breath break. Then, you immediately continue with perhaps a pushup set that lasts another 20 seconds. Then another 10-second break. The 20-second bouts should number 8. You can pick from a variety of high intensity workout bouts that do the job of maxing you out while you perform the Tabata. Other examples (other than the two above) are lunges, squats, burpees and quite a few more. Now, be sure to check trusted sources online for descriptions of the proper ways of performing these exercises (I'll be sure to provide a few of these descriptions myself at some point). Important thing is: you've got to be breathing (and sweating) like you were promised a million big-ones to try to catch up to Usain Bolt without needing to surpass him (you know, at least have him in your sights the entire sprint period, which might prove rather hard to be sure). You find that at the end of a full Tabata, you're so out of breath and fatigued you can't even stand straight. That's the whole idea (wide grin). Question though is, why? Why perform an exercise routine that makes you wonder why you had to do it in the first place as you try to suck in enough air into your lungs to convince yourself you're still alive?

Afterburn.

You're cooking your sunny side up. You flip the sunny side down just after you kill the cooking flame because you know the residual heat in the pan is just enough to form that thin film or coating on the yolk that keeps all the gooey goodness inside (hmm... yummy). Source of the heat is gone. But you still got some heat left to finish off the delectable all-timer. The point (I do love to illustrate, forgive me): when you do HIIT like Tabata, you experience this desirable little phenomenon called 'Afterburn'. Much like the analogy above, the Tabata (HIIT) workout that maxed you out (like the heat that cooked your sunny side) leaves 'residual energy' (as it were) that keeps 'cooking' long after you quit the bout. In other words, after your HIIT routine, your body keeps burning stored forms of energy for hours and hours – even days. In exercise physiology parlance, this 'afterburn' can be termed, Excess Post-Exercise Oxygen Consumption (EPOC). Simply, since your high intensity workout left your body still a tad saturated with wastes like lactic acid, not to mention depleted energy stores, your body's oxygen requirements to facilitate waste removal and replenish depleted energy stores get a significant hike, and your metabolic rate stays elevated long after you quit the HIIT bout. Your brain actually instructs your lungs to increase oxygen intake and corresponding capacity during afterburn. This is so because oxygen is one of your body's essential ingredients in its metabolic processes and, an elevated metabolic rate will translate into a corresponding increase in oxygen consumption, as it should. I should quickly chip this in: your metabolic rate is the rate at which your body converts (or burns) calories to produce energy. Interesting thing is, the afterburn effect carries on even while you're at rest. This 'rest-state' metabolic rate is what is referred to as 'basal metabolic rate' (BMR). So, while the typical HIIT like Tabata truly, fully, sometimes unbearably, exhausts you, the 'afterburn' effects are totally worth it. Your body keeps metabolizing 'calories' (by means of EPOC) stored as glycogen and (oh yes) fat, long after your session ended – up to 72 hours, it is estimated. Plus, you maybe remember when I indicated I was (not a little) averted to long periods of workout regimens - you know, looking to max results in the shortest possible time? The Tabata actually helps you there. If planned well, you not only get to exercise for shorter periods per time, you also get pretty much the same long-term benefits of other less intense, longer bout, exercise regimens.

So, when I mentioned 'Calories' above, did you get it? What are calories? Put quite simply: calories represent units of energy. Or 'latent energy, measured', like I sometimes like to put it. You see, when your body does physical work, it burns or metabolizes stored energy (or calories) to produce the active energy (fuel) needed to perform the needed work. Calories are energy units irrespective of the form the energy sources take. For instance, a burger patty and a cup of cappuccino even though essentially different in nature (one being meat-based protein, and the other a beverage) can both be represented in terms of calories. A typical beef patty, and three cups of cappuccino both contain roughly 200 calories, each. In effect, they both contain sources of energy the body can both store and use, measured in units of calories. When you consume a food item (solid, liquid, and all in-between) containing say 100 calories, it means your body just acquired an additional 'stock' of energy. Like megabytes or gigabytes - as fixed storage - in the computer world, you can either leave the 'stock' of calories (data) unused or, burn (use it) to perform physical work. Now, quite unlike your computer storage that leaves the used data stored even after use (unless deleted) in its physical circuits, the body doesn't leave metabolized calories in its energy storehouses. They stay gone. Point? When you consume high calorie foods and don't burn (or metabolize) them the most you can, they store in your body, initially as glycogen, then (annoyingly) as big bad fat. So, you really don't want to leave those calories lying uselessly around. Computers don't get fat.

So, Tabata? Like other HIIT regimens, the Tabata's afterburn effect keeps metabolizing (or burning) calories up to 72 hours (as indicated above) after the session ended. Now you know why it 'packs a punch'? It has been shown through research that HIIT regimens typically produce more afterburn effects than steady-state cardio routines. And the best part? They take less time.

My Tabata journey comes next.

<u>*"May The Force Be With You"*</u>

Not really a Star Wars fan. *Although I did thoroughly enjoy the oldest releases with Harrison Ford as Han Solo*. However, I *can* identify with some of the essential philosophies and ideals. The famous quote heading this part well, is famous. While the thought here conveyed is that of an unseen universal 'force' that is all-powerful, and all-pervasive (I assume), there is the ever-present theme of: *'Willpower'*. Yep, while Skywalker (and fellow Jedi) could tap into this 'force' at will, the influence here of personal willpower cannot be overstated. To be successful at being a Jedi, you had to have a willpower strong enough to fully harness the (perhaps limitless) powers of 'the force'.

Not a sci-fi fan? The subject of WILL runs through every facet of human life and endeavor. People shot in the head and torso several times and absolutely refused to die; the woman whose child was trapped under a car and willed herself to lift the, perhaps over a ton vehicle off her baby ('hysterical strength'); the 'me' (yours truly) who went learning to swim unattended, unwittingly wondering off into the deep end of the pool, realizing I couldn't feel the pool's smooth flooring but still managing to thrash limbs and all until safe at the side railings. *Had no interest in exiting that early – didn't even have a bucket list yet.*

Martial arts? The examples are endless here. Buddhist/Shaolin monks and their incredible physical feats that really do defy our comprehension; Japanese Kendo masters using katanas to slice through (in full strike motion) watermelons perilously placed on a volunteer's belly, without the slightest break in the skin of the volunteer (blindfolded); trained fists breaking through concrete walls with only slight bruises to show.

***Willpower***.

That's the common thread that runs through all above. It is said that we are only limited by the amount of personal willpower we can summon. Now, while I wouldn't go as far as jumping off the Burj Khalifa, nor recommend doing so (expecting to survive), to test this, it is quite true that we *can* accomplish incredible physical and mental feats as humans when we summon super-powerful, inherent willpower. The examples above, among countless others validate this. I really would have kicked it in that pool many years ago, if I hadn't 'willed' myself to survive. Hadn't learned a thing about how to swim and just wanted to try what I saw on tv on my own. Except that I had no idea there was a deep end in that pool plus, there was no one around to warn, or help, me. When I realized I could actually die (so unceremoniously at that), a survival instinct kicked in that galvanized intrinsic will. I fought. Hard. Thrashing, kicking, whatever I had to do. And, I survived. 'You drown, not by falling into a river, but by staying submerged in it' (Paulo Coelho).

Pretty sure you know where I'm headed with this train. My personal journey to fitness after forty had me digging deep to find a willpower I had somehow left mostly redundant, irrelevant even, as I never really had a cause to actually use it since my pool ordeal. *Had another incident where I absolutely had to summon that will. I'll probably tell later*. By definition, willpower is 'control exerted to do something or restrain impulses' (Oxford). So, you're either actively controlling your thoughts and actions towards accomplishing something palpable, or you're doing so to restrain yourself from acting in an undesirable manner. Either way, there is significant effort in control of your senses.

Brass tacks: Tabata is frigging hard, and I had to summon a willpower, I apparently had, in order to perform 3 full Tabatas 5 days a week. To be sure, I didn't start out that way.

Was already half a month into my intermittent fasting routine when I decided to go the Tabata way to fulfil the exercise element of my fitness goals. Also, at the same time the fasting began (or a few days before), I had started a regimen of spot-jogging, a few lunges and even fewer pushups at least 3 times a week. So, you could consider all that 'pre-Tabata' warmup (perhaps not an actual warmup I know, but it served in my case). And when I got into Tabata per se, I could only do one full one 5 times a week. Didn't take long to ascend to 3 full Tabata's each day five days a week, and I actually managed to sustain that level for a full three months. I wish I could say it got easier and easier. No chance. Thing is, HIITs are *supposed* to max you out. Each time. If a session does not, it simply doesn't cut it.

My slight detour above to the subject of willpower was not discursive.

First time I completed 3 full Tabatas, I had a childhood dream resurface. It was me flying over unnamable land masses, euphoric and madly smug. There was this marked difference though: for the first time in substantive memory, I could actually jet through the clouds, and all around, at fictional speeds. Was never quite able to do that before. My flight dreams hitherto were always… disappointing, because I never could go as fast as I wished. Always this bedeviling, inexplicable, drag. Not this time though. My speed was outstanding (not to mention the typical preternatural strength in attendance). All out of your regular superhero flick, except there was no 'hero-ing' here. Just me enjoying souring through the air at top speeds. Exhilarating to be able to that for the first frigging time. And I had my first successful, 3 full sets of Tabatas to thank for it. You get this feeling like you won the lottery or something bogusly similar when you complete a regimen of Tabatas. Each time. That's how challenging it is. And it is precisely that level of challenge to the body that produces the goods in that ephemeral bout.

So, willpower? You sure do need it to get through each session. You *will* feel like throwing in the towel or raising the white one every so often. I know I did. I dug in again, each time wayward drudgery crept up, or when my 'get-up-and-go' 'got-up-and-left', and found the willpower to persist. You find it always helps to reignite your initial motivation. At the pool, during my near-death brush, survival was all the motivation I needed. *Hadn't even had that first kiss with my crush yet, so no chance I was going out that easy.* And, as far as this journey of mine, the 'catalyst' in the beginning served pretty well as sufficient incentive. It was all too present to miss (how could you not abhor the sight of an obscured crotch), as I drove myself to keep up with the HIIT and, as I gradually got to see (oh joyous) results, motivation more easily swung by.

At this point I need to sound this rather serious caveat: HIIT isn't for everyone!

Even for me, it was rather risky, given my affair with asthma and chronic bronchitis (but I'm stubborn like that). HIIT is NOT the only route to fitness (especially after forty). I'd even go as far as not recommending it at all if you've got any of the conditions above (including some serious cardiovascular problems) and without an appreciable level of fitness beforehand. Simply not advisable. You should CONSULT your doctor if you're plagued (pardon the expression but being a sufferer, it does seem that way) by any of those conditions (or similar) above before ever trying out a HIIT routine. Please! There are other robust, steady-state exercise regimens that do the job just as well. Believe me.

However, my personal journey took me the Tabata way, and that's what this whole 'gig' is about. And, it worked pretty well, with the intended benefit of a much shorter duration, both in terms of per session workouts and, the entire period. There were times I would begin to 'wheeze-up' while doing a Tabata. I would quickly pick up my inhaler and 'drag' during the 10 second rest phase and continue till I completed the entire session. Again, willpower. There's just no getting around it. My asthma eventually 'came around' and began to comply with my wishes. Had fewer and fewer attacks as the Tabatas continued. Fact is, the muscles that help you breathe, as well your lungs get a serious efficiency boost when you regularly exercise, regardless of the regimen path you take.

So how exactly did I perform each Tabata? Is there a correct way to do them? Can a varied approach benefit similarly?

Covid-19.

Around the same time the disease became a pandemic and restrictions were placed where I live, I was only about a week into my *journey*. Now, this would have been a dampener of sorts if I was your typical 'social bee' and needed to hit the gym every time I wanted to work out. Not me. My entire workout regimen was performed in my very own bedroom (well, mine and the missy's), and with practically no equipment.

Here is how it all worked out in my case.

First, I got an app installed on my phone. Pretty nifty one. Designed specifically for Tabata, it times your 20-second sessions with beep sounds to keep you apprised, and then alerts you when your 10-second rest periods are about to start and times that with the associated beep sounds as well. Various other app options allow you to customize your sessions - set how many full Tabata cycles you want to perform per daily session, for instance. You can browse through your app store to choose and install an app that does this. Quite a few out there.

So, armed with my app, I swung right into the my very first Tabata. 'Swung' quite aptly described it, since I never got into any warm-up activity before beginning. That is the general recommendation actually. You really should warm up before beginning any moderate to high-intensity exercise routine. Now, why is that?

If you've largely been sedentary preceding your newfound drive to exercise, you might want to 'ease into' things by subtly 'waking' up your muscles, heart and lungs and preparing them for the work ahead. This process - warm up - helps loosen those stiff joints and flex those tense muscles so they don't get a seriously rude awakening by twisting or tearing when the serious workout starts (and long after it ends – muscle soreness, sprains etc.). Your heart and lungs too get a mild dose of what is to come and get a bit more prepared by increasing blood circulation and oxygen consumption to better handle the impending workload. Your overall metabolism gets a kickstart by increasing just enough to make the tedium ahead not be that much a sharp shoot up. There is still controversy amongst researchers (no surprises there) as to whether warmups actually do prevent injuries, but it is generally considered a good idea to do so pre-workout. What'll hurt?

Never did do any warm up. My bad? But, in my case, I had some years of martial arts training in my younger days to thank for the fact that I didn't get to pay seriously for the omission. At least that's how I figured things. I suppose these early life experiences may count for something after all. I mean, it was a full 20 years since I did any martial arts training before I undertook my recent journey. I guess, in that long, my body still had a 'hangover' from grueling, body-assaulting training sessions. Whatever the case, my skipping warmups and swinging right into full Tabatas didn't take the expected toll. Suffice it to add that I didn't have a serious heart condition that would make doing a Tabata well, strictly a taboo. So, unless you are of the same pedigree as me, you might want to do some warmups before kicking right into the Tabata. Warmups typically include activities as unspectacular as swinging your arms up and then side to side, bending down to touch your toes a few times; even light dancing. No specifics here, just that you want to prep your body by lightly elevating your heart rate, oxygen consumption and muscle-joint flexibility. There's a plethora of suggested warmup activities online. You know the drill: simply type 'warmup exercises' in the address pane of your browser and let your search engine do the work. Averted to the 'www'? Just do some stretching, leg and arm swinging and a bit of brisk walking or light jogging on the spot, and you should be sufficiently warmed up. You should be careful not to overdo it if you're planning on hitting full Tabatas since you already got your work cut out for you in that unforgiving arena.

So, I swung right into sprinting on the spot for my very first 20-second Tabata exercise bout. If you've ever had to do the basic sprint back in your school years, you know this is no 'breezy day Sunday'. You do a spot-sprint by, well, sprinting on the spot. You're raising your knees as high up as you can and moving your arms as you would if you were actually doing the 50/100-meter dash. Except, you're doing it standing in one place. Go ahead, give it a try.

I did that 20-sescond sprint 5 times with 10-second rests between. Sprinted 20 seconds, rested 10 seconds – 5 times. After the first 5 sprints, I felt like I would die. That intense. But the full Tabata wasn't over. I now went down and did pushups for another 20 seconds (fast as I could). It rounded up rather nicely to 20 pushups per 20 second bouts. Next, I threw in some reverse lunges (will describe) for the following 20-second bout. And then I finished up with another 20-second pushup bout. A total of eight, 20-second bouts (a full Tabata). Of course, in between each bout was a 10-second rest period (you find soon enough those rest periods seem wholly insufficient). And so, my first full Tabata was complete. If you're doing more than one, you should space by about 3-4 minutes.

My choice of specific exercises to fill up my Tabata cycle were by no means stochastic though. I chose them for good reason. I'll tell you.

The spot-sprinting for one. It's one very effective workout for the heart and lungs, or 'cardio' - as is most generally used to term these workouts. Whether done lightly, moderately or intensely (as in the case with Tabata), cardio exercises strengthen and improve the capacity of the heart and lungs to perform work. You get the sense of this benefit when you discover you're better able to do physical work with minimal fatigue. There's a marked scaleup in efficiency. And the more, (or harder) the cardio workouts, the better the heart/lung system becomes. It's really a classic case of concomitance in variation relationship. The more intense or profound the cause (cardio exercise), the greater the corresponding effect (improved heart/lung efficiency). Now, this is a key element of physical fitness as, the better your heart and lungs perform, the fitter you are. I didn't just want to lose the belly fat and associated 'hate' handles, I needed to become fitter so I could be better able to handle physical activity, without tiring out so easily. I'm pretty sure you can conjure up in your mind at least one physical activity you would just love to be better at. *My wayward mind certainly can.* So, it made absolute sense (in my case), to make the cardio routine prominent in my lineup of Tabata exercises.

**Don't forget, my composite catalyst at the start had hypertension out front. I did also mention I was asthmatic. These two conditions benefit considerably from cardio workouts. Your heart strengthens and requires less pressure to get the blood out there to other parts of your body. Your lung capacity also ratchets up, making your asthma attacks easier to handle as well as help reduce those episodes. These are significant, tangible benefits that truly justify the means. Caveat: don't you dare try the Tabata if you've got chronic bronchitis or BP in the nether regions of risk. Consult your physician!!!**

The pushups? Well, that's probably a no-brainer. Needed bigger and firmer biceps, triceps, and pecs (chest muscles) to flaunt as evidence of my hard work. Not all ostentation though. Stronger muscles overall make for a more efficient Musculo-Skeletal system. This is never a bad thing. You know this for sure when your better half playfully asks that you carry her full 90 kilograms, for instance. You either take the challenge smiling or you quickly erase any smile you had on before the challenge. Now, this was an actual scenario for me (or one of several). Before my journey my Missy would often quip about how I couldn't even lift her off the ground and yet I claimed to have been into martial arts in my younger days. No sense explaining that that was eons ago because well, she knew that already. So, I would instead summon a strength that was only a shadow of days lofty and far gone, and actually attempt the 'epic' lift. I always did lift her clear off the ground, but for only the briefest moments. Couldn't be briefer. But I had to contend with very unpleasant back and waist strain for days and days after. This made the Missy's torment of me (with hysterical laughter) even more unbearable than the pain.

And then, about only 7 or so weeks into my Tabata routines, and thousands of pushups (perfectly executed I might add) later, the challenge resurfaced. Smile stayed on this time. I always did fancy a chance at testing my 'renewed' strength and stamina. This was it. This time, she stayed suspended (by yours truly) in the air a full minute, and I wasn't about to put her down either. She asked, restrained worry shading her expression, "you going to be okay?". I replied, 'no worries babe, I got this". She had this look of 'measured incredulity' on her face that would have cracked me up if I wasn't so preoccupied with maintaining that pose as long as I could muster. Sort of like that look Lois Lane had on when 'Sups' flew up the Daily Planet tower to rescue his damsel (Lane) who was falling to her demise. He caught her in mid-air, and to Lois' utter disbelief he said, 'it's ok, I've got you'. Lane, with that same look of 'measured incredulity' as with my Missy, would then utter the immortal words, 'You've got me, who's got you!'. That scene always did manage to crack me. Saw that movie with my folks at a cinema those many years ago and it still ranks as one of my all-time favorites (that scene anyway).

So, there it was. My very first successful 'lift'. Didn't get any of that post-ordeal pain in those regions above either. Total win. No gain saying, my wife looked at me different (if not suspiciously) a while beyond that day. I should say though: the goal here isn't to get all brawny like Dwayne J (do pardon the language D.J) and, if you're my age, that may prove especially hard anyway. The real idea: get stronger, get fitter, do better.

As you will get to see soon enough, the pushups weren't the only strength-training workouts I did in the period. But I'll get to that later. This wouldn't be much of an adventure if I gave all the details in one fell swoop would it?

Now, the reverse lunges? I promised to describe this exercise type somewhere above. I prefer to deliver on promises so, here goes.

Lunges (forward or reverse), are a type of workouts that target your knees, thighs, back, and core muscles. They strengthen these joints and muscles, improve your balance and stability, and contribute a great deal to that afterburn effect of HIIT routines we 'talked' about earlier. You can also throw in better posture as additional benefit. You want to stand with hands on your hips and legs hip-width apart. Okay, this starting position isn't strict and all, but it does help to have a consistent starting posture that best helps you to progress into the actual exercise. So, you got the start in the bag. Next, while firming up your core, you take a big step backwards with (first) your left leg – or right - and aim at keeping your upper body straight as you do so (hands on hips help there). Your end position should have your right leg – or left - (which bears the weight of this move) bent at the knee forming a right angle (90 degrees), and your left leg – or right - thrown back also forming that angle but with the knee almost touching the ground. Doesn't matter which leg you initiate with. Now, you can substitute the '90-degree' part above with this: right thigh parallel to the ground, and left thigh perpendicular (or vertical) also to the ground. You then repeat this movement, this time stepping back with the right leg. Do this for 20 seconds, as the Tabata cycle dictates. I sometimes varied my lineup by doing two sets of 20-second reps of the lunges, and adjusted the other routines accordingly. Let me reiterate that you should ensure your upper body remains straight while tightening your core the entire time you engage the movements involved in the reverse lunge. You more fully glean the benefits above when you do.

The internet: oh, how I both love and hate this tool. You really only need to type 'reverse lunges' into the (ever receptive) address pane of your browser *or* 'the tube' and watch as a world of 'how-to' videos hit your senses. Enjoy. Can't go wrong. *Or maybe you could*. Do be circumspect as you search, as you don't want to end up with less than accurate information. So, if what you see demonstrated fits generally with my description above, you should be good.

And now. *Sheepish grin appears*. As far as benefits of lunges? Here goes my absolute favorite (had to give this one its standalone paragraph): you get a significant boost in your sex life when you include lunges in your exercise routines (HIIT and moderate intensity workouts alike). Yup, it's true. This cuts across the gender divide as well. An uncle of mine actually first gave me this hint (he made it sound more like absolute truth though), and I consequently gave it the 'scrub' through research. Turns out you're better able to perform 'fantasy' positions when you strengthen the areas of the body that lunges target. Additionally, it is believed that your 'area' (if you're male) gets improved blood supply, and that gives you the type of 'boner' you can smile about. You can also throw into the cocktail the fact that you get to last longer between the sheets (or mostly above, if you're like me). See now why I just had to give this a whole, juicy, paragraph? So, learn to do lunges correctly and enjoy all of the, oh so, 'glorious' benefits.

Of all the activities I did during my journey, the Tabata was easily the hardest and most challenging. It was also one of the most beneficial. You just feel that your body got a fitness make-over. Everyday tasks that previously proved testy just get a tad seamless as you perform them. It's not a feeling you can miss or ignore. It's just so, open-and-shut.

Keep this little bit in mind: you can vary the intensity of your HIIT workouts depending on your body's capacity at that particular time. The important thing is to stick to the 20-10-second work/rest cycle of 8 in total (in the case of Tabata), and work yourself the hardest you can, without passing out in the process. You know a successful HIIT set when you're markedly out of breath, are sweat drenched, and generally feel like you maybe barked up the wrong tree. Feel your body as you go along and vary how hard you work without compromising the goal of maxing yourself out. As you progress with the Tabata, you soon find that your body is adapting to the significant work done and almost seems to beg for more, more, more. You make sure to give it. Now, this only translates into more rigorous 20-second bouts and the usual 10-second rest periods in attendance. The entire workout period of 4 minutes remains unchanged. A Tabata newbie and a veteran will both spend 4 minutes total, each, but will be worlds apart as far as workout intensity. So, work within your 'range' of capacity and observe how your body builds strength and endurance as you go along.

You might also want to keep focused during your sessions, as distractions don't work too well. It's just four minutes you know. One time, my two-year-old boy (we nicknamed him 'warrior' for his tirelessness at play, and 'fight') barges in on me while I perform a Tabata, takes one look at his daddy sprinting madly in one spot and decides to rush in and grab a hold of his legs (not sure what went through his mind, but he maybe wanted to give a go at rescuing his old man – or something). Had to give pause to the whole workout set. Started all over – not ideal at all, considering it's hard enough doing a full Tabata without distractions. So, keep distractions at bay while you 'work it'. 'Warrior' met a locked door the next time he came hoping to barge in. Of course, working out at a gym is a whole different scenario. Still, you don't want to be too mindful of that hot female with unbelievable curves working out near you. Keep focused. Get it done. Fraternize all you want afterward. Remember: Tabata is a time-based routine, and missing your work/rest cues don't lend well to the expected results.

So, how might you navigate a Tabata workout routine at a gym? I didn't go the gym path in my journey, true (being an incurable introvert and all, except when I drink and transform to the ultimate social beast), but I did promise to teach a thing or two as you came on this journey with me. So, if you absolutely must be around fellow fitness seekers (and 'showboaters' alike) and do hit the gym, here are a few pointers.

The bicycle Ergometer. This is one of three gym tools you might find especially useful in fulfilling the demands of a typical Tabata. Might be interesting to note that this was pretty much the tool Izumi Tabata (Ph.D.), who created the whole routine, used in his research that produced the wonderful results that constitute the Tabata HIIT variant. It's also called the 'stationary bicycle' since well, it's fixed to the floor. You also got these fancy digital displays near the handles up front that do all sorts of useful stuff like time your workout period - which feature you absolutely require for a successful Tabata.

So, get on a stationary bike and put the pedals to work! Start leisurely to fulfill the 'warmup' ideal and to get a feel of what is to come. A minute or two should do nicely. Then, ride as hard as you can! Imagine you're trying to outrun the devil and you got only that bike. You get the idea. 20 seconds. Rest 10 seconds. Repeat 8 times. Four minutes total. One full Tabata in the bag.

The Elliptical machine. I'd be hitting this one regularly If I was the gym sort. The elliptical machine really does 'bring it'. Your arm, leg, core, and back muscles all get the treatment with this gym equipment. Various settings enable you increase or decrease resistance to both the arm and leg movements as you work the handles and pedals, monitor speed, and accurately time your workout. You 'work' the pedals by pushing them with your feet in a forward motion; the handlebars by pulling and pushing on them with your hands, alternating. Doing a workout on the elliptical often resembles running and really does deliver similar effects and more. When you tighten your core muscles (remember the 'core' refers mostly to the abdominals, lower back and pelvic muscles) as you work, you benefit as this action helps increase your core strength and improves posture and stability, which effects may otherwise be compromised since you have handlebars to hold for support; although you could try working the pedals without using the handlebars to further build core strength. You might want to start slow as warmup, working the legs first while holding the stationary bar (there's typically one) with both hands, and then transiting to the dynamic handlebars when comfortable (if you're a newbie). Now, ramp things up as you start the Tabata. The warmup helps you get the feel of the elliptical if you're new to it, as well as provide the usual benefit of preparing your body for the hard stuff coming. Remember to hit the timer when about to start the Tabata session and restrict work to the 20-10-second work/rest cycle. So: you work as hard and as fast as you can on the pedals and handles for 20 seconds; hold the stationary bar as you cease work for the following 10 seconds; restart timer for the next 20—10-second cycle, and then repeat another seven times to complete a full Tabata. Peachy. Do remember to push hard enough to get your rate up and about without giving yourself a seizure. Quit it if things get testy the first time. But don't give up overall. Your body soon gets used to the new picture you're painting and responds accordingly.

In no time, you will be doing one full Tabata with the attendant exhaustion, yes, but with a sensation that is unmistakably an awareness of a new capacity to switch things up a notch to two full Tabatas. And then perhaps, even three. Not a pipe dream - although it would certainly feel like it the first few times; a (not whimsical) three full Tabatas really is the potential if you persist. Again, the internet is replete with videos and how-to information regarding the elliptical. Do gorge, if you feel the need to. When and if you do hit the gym for this workout and others, hopefully you will find additional help in the gym instructors (where available and sufficiently competent), and be properly guided. Nevertheless, there should be enough above to get you started on your own if you choose to go it alone. And oh, don't get off the elliptical until the pedals have completely come to a stop. Could get a tinge nasty.

The Treadmill. No gym isn't worth it's designation as such without a treadmill (or so it appears). The 'mill' is engineered to drive you to your absolute maximum or, simply to engage you in more leisurely exercise strides. You get to choose your preferred outcome. For the Tabata, using a treadmill can get a bit tricky and would require that you exercise the utmost caution. The 'www' is overabundant with the infamous 'gym fails' line of videos that feature the treadmill in some rather serious mishaps. So, unless you want to earn your fame (hardly any fortune) by suffering some opprobrium, you want to be careful with this gym staple. Here again, the warmup is recommended to get you all fired up for the Tabata. Just take a leisurely stroll on the mill and let your metabolism get the message it's about to get some 'heat'. Then, holding the handlebars for support, step onto the side panels that don't move, straddling with both feet; set to sprint (don't forget to monitor the timer for the 20-second bout), control your breathing, then step on the fast-moving rollers (still holding the handles); get your balance and then let go of the bars. 20 seconds. Step off to the side panels when the 20 seconds are up. You know the drill: 20-10-second work/rest cycle. Eight times for the full Tabata. The sprint setting on most treadmills are variable depending on your level of fitness and experience (not to mention gusto). Find a setting above average that works you to the max. That's the whole point of the Tabata, remember? Feel free to do that online thing again – plenty videos on there that show you what to expect and proper form to take.

There you go. Three, sparkling, equipment-based Tabata workouts you can do at the gym (hopefully safely). If you get to the point of blasting off more than one full set, you can switch tools by using any one of the three suggestions above. So, say you started on the stationary bike, you could do the next full set on maybe the elliptical; and then (if you're blissfully suicidal like yours truly), hop onto the treadmill for the final run (if three full Tabatas is your aim). Remember to space full sets by 3-4 minutes so your body recovers some - even if not sufficiently - in between sets.

So, gym freak, you're done with the Tabata. Cool down. Now this is an actual activity that has nothing to do with downing a cold beverage or chilly water. The post-workout cooldown is the recommended way to end any moderate to high-intensity workout and is quite beneficial. The crux is that a cooldown helps restore your body's natural physiological balance after your intense workout which put a ton-load of stress on your vital systems like your heart, lungs, muscles and joints. You want your heart rate and blood flow nearly back to pre-workout levels before you carry on with regular activity as this helps your recovering muscles (heart inclusive) restore to a state they are able to function normally. Breathe deeply to get as much oxygen into your lungs for delivery to your fatigued muscles. There are several suggested cooldown activities that help your post-Tabata, stressed-out body get back to some semblance of normalcy. Expectedly, they are easy to perform and aim to coax your body to relax and try to forget you almost got it thrashed. The basic ones include simple stretches. Easy as sitting on the floor and pulling your knees up, and then stretching your legs out again a couple or more minutes. Or simply jog lightly, or walk briskly (at first), and then leisurely. Really that easy, although there are more than a dozen different cooldown activities. Choose which best suits you. Yes, the web again. Getting old? Just type 'cooldown exercises' and wait for it.

If you used any of the three gym tools above for your Tabata however, your cooldown could be as seamless as dialing down to the barest minimum on workout intensity. Riding the stationary bike, for instance, would simply require that you pedal less intensely after your full Tabata set reducing gradually till you're just riding leisurely without the 'devil' in pursuit. The treadmill offers much the same luxury of seamless transition from high-intensity to cooldown. Simply step onto the side panels and set the mill to light jogging or brisk walking, get back on and work yourself down to a leisurely stroll.

You already know my Tabata journey didn't take me anywhere near the gym and of course, Covid-19 wasn't to blame. You also probably remember I never did fancy doing any warmups before my workouts. The cooldown though?

You guessed it! Zip. Didn't do that either (sheepish grin again). Not that I have a penchant for the antithetical, it's just well, yes maybe I do. It's mostly instinct though. I just never a saw a need to warm up or cool down during my Tabata journey. My body simply didn't dictate as much. Didn't experience anything adverse either (also, there is no definitive research that has shown that cool-downs are requisite as part of your total workout routine). However, that was me. I do recommend that you follow the suggestions regarding warmup and cooldown as you embark on your own journey to fitness, if you so decide. They really do help prepare your body pre-workout, and then relax you afterward.

Ever heard of **mountain climbers**? Now here is one workout that does wonders for your core muscles while delivering the intensity required for the Tabata. It's one of many exercises that burn belly (and indeed total body) fat. The reason I singled this one out of the many 'belly-buster' exercises is because I included it in my Tabata sets when I decided to add a little 'spice' to my lineup. Depending on how I felt at the moment, I swiped one or two routines out of my regular with the mountain climber. So, I had my spot-sprinting; pushups; lunges; and then the mountain climbers forming my lineup eventually. This combo worked quite well for me and my set goals. Four key areas: the cardio-respiratory system comprising mainly the heart, associated blood vessels, and lungs; upper body muscles ('pecs' or chest, and arm muscles); core muscles; lower body (leg muscles), all get worked with the Tabata. The result is that your body's capacity to do physical work, its fat burning processes (even at rest – afterburn), and general fitness, all get a significant boost. Did I mention your psyche also gets the work-over as your fitness level increases, shooting up your confidence and improving your general state of mind? Each time you work out, your brain releases 'happy-you' chemicals like 'endorphins' and 'dopamine' which, yes, make you happy. You get a mood swing-up hours after your workout. Totally worth it. I know I already enumerated these key benefits somewhere earlier, but it really never gets old. And, as you begin to experience them yourself, your sense of accomplishment rises, even as the Tabata (and indeed all HIIT) scares the hell out of you occasionally when you're gasping for air after full sets (there were times I wondered if the full sets of Tabata I just concluded might be the end of me). It's absolutely okay to 'freak out' sometimes from sheer exhaustion after your intense workout. For me, those moments only reinforced my confidence I had just completed a damned successful Tabata routine. Very fleeting though, those feelings. Seconds even, and you soon feel like all is right again with the universe.

The mountain climbers? I believe a brief description might suffice. The reason it's called that is not farfetched, since the appearance while performing one is of climbing something, except the 'something' here is the floor. Even as you're not pulling your weight up against gravity compared to when doing actual vertical climbing, the mountain climber provides just enough resistance to produce similar results. So, you assume a position on the floor as if you want to start pushups with your body raised, arms extended, and palms flat on the floor. This start position also resembles another core/upper body exercise called the **plan.** Steady yourself, then just 'climb' the floor by simulating the movements of actual climbing; pulling one knee up towards your chest with toes of that leg pointing towards the floor but not touching (the other leg stays put for support); repeat movement with other leg, alternating both in quick succession and just - climb that floor! 20 seconds (for the Tabata).

When introducing the Tabata, I know I gave a short list of possible workouts to include in your HIIT lineup. There are over a dozen in fact, and you'll probably come across names like burpees, jumping jacks, squat jacks, jump rope, and many others. Experiment as much as you like and find the right combo for YOU. If it helps you to have a fixed set of exercises in your lineup, create one and stick to it. Of course, you *could* also vary that set using any of the long line of possible exercises to fill your lineup. But do ensure you've mastered (or at least be reasonably proficient at performing) the one or more exercises you want to vary your lineup with before doing the actual routine. This is vital because doing exercises right - during a high intensity bout like the Tabata - will go a long way in preventing possible injury, as well as help ensure the realization of the desired results. A few practice sessions should hit the mark in this regard.

So sad. We're going to have to leave sweet, sweet Tabata in peace for now, before I become guilty of blatherskite (not that that bothers me much).

My journey with the routine took me to heights (and depths) I wasn't aware I could once again reach. I dove down deep into my psyche, found a willpower I thought had long deserted me, and pulled it right out of those 'forbidden' recesses of my mind; made it go to work for me. I lost a full 12 kilograms (and a fraction) in 12 weeks. My 'love to hate' handles completely disappeared and, finally, I could look down and find my 'crotch' looking right back, and I didn't have to bend or strain to see my old buddy, in all its glory. I lost much undesirable fat and gained lean muscle in all the right places. Libido, and associated sexual prowess (in *my* case), was sufficiently restored, and the missy still lives in mild shock. Best of all, I found a physical capacity long lost. Every physical effort just seemed a whole lot less of an effort. Felt like I could do anything!

But don't you think for even a micro-second this journey is over. Intermittent fasting, Tabata, and the all-important willpower didn't do it all for me.

So far, I hope you could gather a few useful items to include in your souvenir holder as we take the next wondrous step in this journey of mine you so graciously came with me on. And, as you do......'may the force be with you'.

# **_Battle of The Core_**

Sounds straight out of a sci-fi flick.

No connection though. Remember the whole 'catalyst' thing from the get-go, the 'big bang' incentive, that (not so little) spark that lit up the string of events that ultimately led to this journey of mine so far? Wasn't it that abominable, abdominal fat (and associated 'love to hate' handles) that annoyingly obscured view of my genitals without using a mirror? The catalyst.

In exercise physiology/physical fitness parlance, the 'core' refers to the muscles of the abdominal area, lower back, pelvic area and hips, the spine (extending from the base of the head to the pelvis), and the diaphragm (the muscle just beneath the lungs that controls breathing). Although the revered 'six pack' is located in this region, it forms only a part of the entire group of muscles constituting the core. A bit of anatomy here won't hurt one bit (you get to reel out fancy terms when talking about your own journey to fitness). There's the **_rectus abdominis_**. This is that part of your (wishful) six-pack that runs vertically along the middle of your abdomen (in well-defined sections if you're a six 'pack' member), and lends it that name. The rectus abdominis muscle is actually a pair, parallel to each other and divided into eight sections – four on both sides of the abdominal midline. So, on either side of the midline are four sections each of the rectus and the midline separator here is fibrous connective tissue called the **_linea alba_**. The typical six-pack will manifest six sections of the **_rectus abdominis_** and not the actual eight. The lowest pair sort of sinks into the pelvic area and not visible. Lateral to the **_rectus,_** on both sides is the **_transversus abdominis_** which runs horizontally (hence the 'transversus') on both sides of the **_rectus abdominis_**. The pair of rectus and transversus form the most recognizable part of the core. The point of this anatomy lesson? Shrug. Thought it might prove insightful, given the otherworldly attention the 'pack' gets.

The 'pack' was never my mission though. I really, really, really wanted to get rid of unwanted fat in all the wrong places. _That_, was my mission. Of course, in doing so, all the lofty benefits of gaining a good measure of physical fitness, came accompanying.

But, in getting rid of all (or most) of the unsavory fatty deposits in my middle, I needed to build lean abdominal muscle to fortify my core area. A strong, or stronger core is essential to the execution of every day movements, and tasking activities are less daunting. There's a reason the core is called the 'core'. The core of any physical structure lends that system balance, stability; a sturdy, central point from which other extending parts can draw support. The benefits of strengthening the core are quite impressive. You got lower back pain from poor posture? Make the core stronger. You feel you can do better at salsa – strengthen the core. Fact is, any physical activity that involves the coordinated use of your limbs depends on the core to get the job done efficiently. A weak core detracts from this. Bending to pick something up from the floor may seem rather mundane, but for someone with a weak core, it could be quite strenuous. And don't even get me started on how a stronger core can improve your intimate sessions.

So, I knew my two-pronged assault on my body fat (intermittent fasting and the Tabata) was going to blast off on the adipose in short order, but I also needed a stronger core with better toned muscles to replace the distasteful folds in my abdomen. How to do this. 'The battle', next.


### The Chosen Five


Didn't pick that title lightly - Battle of the Core. There really was some battle here. Doing three full Tabatas was grueling enough. Deciding to add a string of core-centric workouts to deal with the 'vacuum' left after diminishing belly fat was, well, maybe stretching it a bit. Still, I did do it. Turned out to be much less daunting as perhaps anticipated.

I chose five specific abdominal exercises for this battle. Process didn't require that much deliberation to be sure. It was mostly a case of what felt right and comfy, yet delivering. The chosen five: **leg drops**; **the plank**; **reverse crunches**; the **reach through crunch**; **bicycle cross crunches**.

Played out thus.

**Leg Drops.** This one is as simple as they get, to describe. Simply lie flat on the ground, legs together not splayed, and arms stretched out on both sides. You should roughly resemble a 'T' when done positioning. I recommend that palms be laid flat on the ground in this position (a bit of twisting here), as this helps to support your core when performing this exercise. Try assuming this pose a sec. Got it? Now, just raise both legs, in tandem, till they're perpendicular (forming a right angle/ vertical) to the ground. I bet now you get why those palms are facing down. Lower the legs and repeat 20 times. The leg drop just dropped. First few times for me didn't cut it. Could only manage 10-15 successful drops. My core caught up eventually, and doing 20 per session actually became breezy.

How did I manage to squeeze in ab exercises with the killer Tabata already, 'killing'? Well, I waited a full 5 minutes after my three full Tabata sets before getting into the abdominal crunches. I figured my body was already all primed up, so why not? Worked pretty. It was all quite seamless. Not a rule though. You may space your routines more than I did and get same or similar results. You could, for instance, do the ab workout set several hours later; or even on a day-on/day-off basis. For me, the leg drops dropped like that – as described.

As you perform this, you just feel your abdominals getting the workout. You're without a doubt those particular muscles are being engaged. That's a good thing. The leg drops are an excellent way to strengthen the core and build abdominal muscle you can actually flaunt.

My battle of the core began with these 'drops'. Every day I did them, along with the four others accompanying. Yes, those four come next.

The **Plank.** A popular one, this. It's one of many exercises termed 'static', since it doesn't involve any dynamic movement. You simply assume a position, and then hold it for a specific period. How to do the plank? Peachy. You do know the regular pushups, right? Position your body as you would one half of a typical pushup when your body is raised above the ground, arms stretched with palms and toes touching the floor and supporting your body's weight. Then hold it. Don't go down, but do look down if you must. Arms straight, your trunk down the legs inclined but straight (your buttock area should slightly jut). Draw your navel inward, tightening your abdominals as you do. And then, count at least 20 seconds (if you can manage it), holding that pose. There are variations to this basic pose and you can explore these online to find one that's agreeable. Your core muscles firm up as you do this exercise and you just know they're working to keep you in that position. That's the whole idea. Fret not if 20 seconds the first time didn't happen. The next couple times should swing you right into that zone. I ended up doing 40 seconds per plank, effortlessly. You do need to space each ab exercise in your lineup by about 10-15 seconds on the average. That amount of time is typically adequate for your muscles to get a quick 'reset' before the next set of exercise-type repetitions (reps).

**Reverse crunches.** There *is* the 'traditional crunch', but that has long been dethroned as part of the ruling class of abdominal workouts. You risk injury for one, plus, the benefits are far too minimal to be worth the fair amount of strain to your lower back (especially). Don't confuse the forward crunch with sit-ups. The traditional forward crunch does not involve lifting your lower back completely off the ground as you execute each crunch. That part of your body stays grounded the entire time. Your upper body lifting only, instead, supplies the resistance the abs require to get activated. Doing the traditional crunch in reverse, however, delivers quite the effect. Your major core muscles are more efficiently engaged, with minimal risk of injury. Particularly, the rectus abdominis (six-pack), and another key core muscle called the ***external oblique*** (along both sides of the abdomen) get some serious activation here. You get stronger, sexier looking abs when you include the reverse crunches in your lineup of core exercises. To be sure, all five of the core exercises in review here deliver similar results, but in varying degrees. You get a sense of how much the core muscles are activated by each exercise type, in the way your core area feels after you perform each of them, and indeed how easy or hard it was to do them.

I found the reverse crunches very much like the name suggests. I could feel my rectus abdominis muscles literally being 'crunched'. To put this another way, it felt like my abdominal innards were being mercilessly compressed; 'juiced'. That considerable tightness felt is unmistakable, if done right. A tad (actually more than a tad) uncomfortable first few times you engage your abs in this way, especially if you're a beginner. But, as is typical of most exercise routines you persist in; it does get easier each time. That 'crunch' feeling never completely goes away though, and that really is the whole point. You're confident your abs are getting the treatment when you feel that tightness. Start with 10, properly executed crunches and then increase as your fitness level inspires.

Ten repetitions of the reverse crunches, done twice - totaling 20 with the usual 10-15-second rest - did it for me. Now tell me, doesn't the fact that each workout set in my core exercises regimen space out each by 10-15 seconds sound a lot like the Tabata? Not in the same ball park I assure you. While both regimens require short rest periods in-between each exercise set, the ab regimen doesn't max you out in the process. The Tabata is designed (and does indeed play out that way) to drive your energy metabolism to its near critical limit. The abdominal workout regimen does not. Ab exercises are mainly designed to strengthen your core muscles (aesthetics too, for the showoffs), not give your heart and lungs a serious shake-up.

So, how to do reverse crunches? Quite a few variations here. Many involve lifting the hips clear off the ground producing a more profound 'crunch' effect by engaging the core muscles more intensely. I went for the more subtle variation however, but 'subtle' here nowhere near undercuts its effectiveness I assure you.

The full reverse crunch: Lie on your back, knees drawn up so your feet are flat on the ground, thighs perpendicular to the floor. Your knees should be bent at a 90-degree angle here. Next, firm up your core, and with arms stretched out on either side of the trunk, palms flat on the floor, slowly raise both legs so your knees reach up and towards your chest as possible, lifting your hips clear off the ground in the process. keep this positions a couple or so seconds. Then, lower legs (and hips) slowly, keeping knees bent as in the starting position. Repeat movement, forming repetitions 8-12 times per set.

Did you notice when I indicated above the main movements be done slowly? For good reason. You want your abdominal muscles doing the task here of lifting and lowering your legs and hips off the ground by sheer force of contraction. You don't get this effect if you use the momentum from a faster execution of the full crunch to pull your knees up towards your chest.

Momentum is what you get when you apply enough force to a motion that is cyclic or continuous. Much like when you're cycling and your initial intense pedaling provides just enough sustained force to keep the pedals rolling without you needing to preserve that initial force. Momentum. You don't want that doing the crunches. Instead, you want your core muscles providing and sustaining the contractile force needed to complete the exercise.

A final note: as you engage your core in the upward and inward (towards chest) movement of your knees, endeavor to breathe out or exhale deeply, as you do that move. Conversely, breathe in deeply as you lower your legs and hips back to starting position. Why the yoga-like routine? Generally, when doing core exercises, it is the standard practice to fully exhale (in slow, deliberate fashion where possible) while contracting the ab muscles. When relaxing those muscles, a full inhalation should accompany. Your core muscles are better activated and engaged when the lungs are emptied of air and ribcage is down. Exhale fully now if you can and observe how your chest appears to compress downwards and inwards, as your lungs release gas within. In this position, your core muscles are unencumbered by pressure in your thorax (chest area) when otherwise filled with air, and are more able to contract efficiently. That's what you want: better, more efficient core-muscle contractions to build strength and engender greater stability in that region and the entire body. When releasing the main contractions in the ab area, in the return movement back to start position doing the crunch, you then inhale deeply and completely. Try inhale that way now as well and observe how your chest area expands, filing your lungs with air. You want to make sure not to push your chest and abdomen out as you do. Your ribcage and core area should expand outwards to the sides (laterally) as you take in air. As I mentioned, key abdominal muscles in the core are better activated and engaged when, breathing during crunches (and other core workouts), is processed this way.

Practice at rest and while exercising to get the hang of this. The benefits are worth the 'tai chi' appearance.

I didn't do the full crunch. Decided to keep the hips planted on the floor while drawing knees and legs as far in towards my chest as would keep the 90-degree knee-to-lower leg angle intact. Completely allowed. Still qualifies as a reverse crunch and is my typical recommendation to start this way and later graduate to executing the fuller 'cousin' as your core becomes stronger. Why did I stay the 'half reverse crunch' lane? Just felt right not to push it. I did have other routines in my lineup, and the famed six-pack musculature just wasn't a goal for me.

So, keep the hips down - if you choose to go my route, as you curl up from the start position of the full reverse crunch. Remember the start position here? It's when you're simply lying on your back with knees drawn up so your feet are flat on the ground; palms also flat on the floor with hands on either side of the trunk (no specific angles here, just ensure hands are placed far enough from the body to supply the needed support for the crunch). Then, as you exhale completely (remember slowly), pull knees up and in towards the chest as far in as possible, but keeping angle between knees and lower legs at 90 degrees (or nearly so). Hips should remain on the floor the entire time. Don't forget: no momentum. Then, breathing in with the same deliberation as with the exhalation, slowly release the core crunch as you return your legs back to the start position; feet flat on the floor with knees bent.

10 reps, done twice (2 sets) settled the half reverse crunch for me. Moving on.

The **Reach through Crunch.** An excellent follow up to the reverse crunch this was for me. Transiting from the 'half reverse crunch' to this just seemed the natural progression. Looks bewitchingly easy to do, but nope. Again, first few times are the pang. Gets easier. Execution? Lie on your back (getting old?) with your knees drawn up so your feet are flat on the floor. Your legs should be separated just enough to allow you 'reach through' with your hands. You want to tighten your core muscles as usual to actively engage them, and as you exhale, reach through your separated legs with both hands (keeping arms straight, still with one hand above the other) just enough so the entire hands and part of the lower arms just beyond your wrists, go completely through; lower back remains on the floor. Inhale completely as you return to starting position, and repeat as many times as your, perhaps now warmed up, abs will allow. Aim at 10 reps to begin with, and ratchet up as you go. Note that when you stretch through both arms with hands above each other in that way above, while you perform the reach through, your core is actively involved here again to sustain the movement of those hands all the way between the legs. This active engagement of the core area muscles, with minimal risk of injury, is what makes the reach through, and other core-centric workouts (that offer same level of safety) so, so worth the effort. So, why not? Do the reach through and, well-toned abs that provide the strength, stability and support your entire body could certainly use, may just well be within your 'reach'.

Wasn't okay with a single set of the reach-throughs, me. Did two sets of 15 each. Typically - first time - I couldn't do 10 successful reaches, much less do a double set. And, reaching my hands all the way through seemed like a bit of a 'stretch'. Core soon caught up with the program and 'reaching through' became quite the cinch. When I felt particularly herculean, I 'reached' for up to 25 reps per set. Totally achievable, believe it.

And now, finally, the **Bicycle Cross Crunches**. First time I saw this, it was quite the surprise: an over-fifty-year-old, very fit looking, definitive (if not starkly six) pack, exuberant man was performing it. If I was looking for excuses not to pursue fitness after forty, that man certainly smashed them up 'real' good. 'I could look like that', I thought. And look so, so, nearly like that I *did*. Don't know how long he'd been at it. Didn't much care. It took *me* three months.

And now, my final core exercise. The bicycle cross crunch, while related to those air cycling moves my 74-year-old mum still does (rather admirably too), is one superb ab workout excellent for delivering the expectations of any core-centric routine. Interesting to note that the cross crunches can also produce the heart-pounding, lung-tasking, body-thrashing effects of the Tabata, if you so desire to have it included in your HIIT regimen. It very much leans towards the 'whole body' workout arena where, your limbs, core, upper body, and your cardio-respiratory system all get worked in one fell swoop. Neat eh? I just love when one action capably produces multiple, desirable effects.

So, this cycle cross crunches - how to do them? You get a little flummoxed first few reps, but no more. I would think it's because of the alternating movements of upper and lower limbs that do require some concerted effort at coordination. Super quick to catch up. And yes, momentum. You want to disregard the momentum 'taboo' when doing reverse crunches; definitely need momentum for this one. Lie on your back (not getting old?) flat, so your lower back does not naturally arch relative to the floor; your knees bent and feet flat on the floor. Place both hands lightly behind your head without opposing fingers touching and, curl (raise) your upper body so your shoulders are slightly off the ground. Raise both legs so your thighs are perpendicular (or at right angles) to the floor, your lower legs parallel to the ground.

What you got is the starting pose. Gets groovy next. Exhale in proper ab workout form, as you now draw one leg-knee in towards your trunk and meet that knee with the opposite arm elbow; the other leg stretches completely out while you do this (although there are variations here). Switch legs and repeat movement touching the other knee with the opposite arm elbow. Start slowly, then build momentum by 'pedaling' in the movements described, alternating legs and elbows. Hands placed lightly behind head and torso raised, help produce much of the crunch effect here as the core muscles are engaged to keep you in this position while the legs, arms and elbows work. You soon note that while alternating legs and elbows, your torso rotates. Be careful not to pull your head up and forward in an effort to ensure your elbows touch the knees. This 'effort' will only end up straining your neck with possible injury. Aim instead at engaging your torso enough to accomplish the rotation required without straining your neck. Your hips should also remain unmoving while the torso does this rotation. Doing this exercise properly ensures you glean the maximum benefits of an effective core workout without (rather common) injury.

Typically, there are variations to cycle cross crunches and you can look these up online (go www!). However, one basic form described above should suffice to set you off nicely.

It's absolutely imperative that you not begin any core-centric exercise routine if you've got neck/back issues – especially if chronic. If you're not sure if you can or can not, do consult a/your physician for proper guidance. You really don't want the title of this part - **battle of the core** - to quite literally translate into 'battle-like' troubles with your spine from improperly executed core workouts. This really isn't a suggestion. Pray heed!

I crushed all the 'crunches' above, and then some. Was nowhere near peachy, I (relentlessly) assure you. My journey took me to, and through, places I'd never before traversed. I repeatedly had to summon uncommon will to drive my lofty ambitions. My personal core battle did its duty. In the three months my journey took, I had an abdomen almost completely bare of undesirable adipose. I also (ecstatically) began to show those fabled signs of a 'packy'. First time I actually saw long-lost definitions along my rectus abdominis, I almost orgasmed from sheer delight. It was still a couple light years from the real-deal six pack, but the sweet lines where there. All that hard work validated. Sublime.

What comes next?

Do follow along now.

***Journey's End?***

## *The Grey, and the Caveat*

Oh, sweet, sweet, science.

Such formidable body of knowledge centuries in building. All the good accomplished by perhaps this most impressive of all human endeavors, took a most rigorous process of testing, testing, and even more testing, through strictly guided research by multiple scientists over many, many decades, before even the simplest scientific fact could be established. It is why you can pretty much rely on science to deliver the goods in daily problem solving. Perhaps the most prominent in this regard is the world of health, medicine and wellness.

In the fitness arena (a subset of health and wellness), there is never-ending research and testing to provide more and more refined guidelines for a better, fuller life. Here, as in all of science, there are established facts and there are the theories and hypotheses that still require more substance to become fully established.

And then……there are the 'grey areas'.

This is how *I* like to describe those rogue phenomena that don't exactly follow established scientific norms. World is full of them. Nope, not going *there.* I will however share one in particular.

One curious one.

You remember that 'composite catalyst' from the get-go? And no, not referring to the bathroom incident. The hypertension.

My blood pressure range was well within the 'do be really, really careful' sort. I had no business doing three full Tabata's encumbered by blood vessels that could very well do without that much pressure. But I did them anyway. Even worse was the fact that I swung right into things without any significant, gradual, buildup.

Also, the asthma. When I got attacks, they came fast, hard. In this regard also, I should've been wary of any physical activity that would strain my lungs enough to trigger an attack, or make one even worse. Still, I pressed on.

I *am* still alive. Healthier than ever. Living with that bothersome trio of ailments (add chronic bronchitis) should have gone the mile as disincentive. Didn't even go one inch.

***The caveat.***

You really don't want to test the limits of your capacity as I did; pursuing fitness after forty. Even as *I* succeeded, it is *not* the norm, especially given my peculiarities. This was all *my journey.* You really must find your own path.

Test your limits by all means. But don't *test* the test. Learn your body enough to know when to quit it. Or slow down.

As a general principle, if you got one or more conditions similar to mine, you should consult your doctor before embarking on your own fitness-after-forty journey. This precaution saves you all of the troubles you might run into diving headlong into any fitness regimen you choose to adopt. This is no joke. Hence the *'caveat'.*

No need to flog this one.


***Chaos, but….***

So, right about now most people on planet earth already think of the year 2020 as the worst in recent history.

Can't argue the prominence of Covid-19 in all of this: a world consumed by a virus that cares very little about anything else than, well, consuming lives; a world mutated from its normal state into this 'grotesque' form unrecognizable on most fronts.

Dissent and protests in previously reticent populations. Social institutions and norms turned essential aberrations. Who would have thought?. Powerful nations split right down the middle in ideology, with latent chaos breathing heavily beneath filmy restraints.

One wonders whether really only an 'extinction level event' (ELE) will awaken humanity to the need to stick prejudices where they belong and just frigging work together for the common good.

And, in the thick of it all…. also, some good.

A landlord dismisses his tenants' rent this year (yes, 2020) to alleviate hardship; an innovative, 'groundbreaker' teacher wins an international award and 1 million dollars in prize money, and decides to share half of it with his losing running mates; the millions of health workers world-wide who daily 'give it all' (even as they watch many in their care take their dying breaths each day) and still, ever so selflessly, continue to fight to put a rampaging pandemic under some measure of control.

There is still some good in this world. Worth holding on to.

2020?

Wasn't all that bad.

My journey did start this same, 'sinister', year. It's taken me on a coaster ride of self-discovery and personal development. And I'm not done yet.


***Journey's End?***


Bear with me now, while I take you through a slight detour; it leads, I assure you.

I always *was* fascinated by martial arts. I was 10 when I got a glimpse of what that world could offer to someone, 'circumstantially' introverted, insecure, and who thought he needed some edge (if only physical, in my eyes) as, perhaps, compensation for perceived deficiencies.

It was this space samurai series I chanced upon when holidaying with some aunts in Paris mid-eighties. I got so enthralled by the combat antics of the show's protagonist while engaging mechanical, alien fiends - in space! His undeniably Japanese pride, cinematic prowess, and brevity in using his combat methods to defeat any foe - and his invariable successes doing so - intrigued me immeasurably. I was young but mostly hardly impressed by anything. But that show did a number on me. Was only there in France a couple months or less, but I took away a lifetime of change. Didn't have that show airing back home, and I *did* search (or had my folks do the dirty work as much as they would pretend to indulge). But I saw enough back in the French capital to do some pretty wild stuff, later. Till this day, I still search the endless depths of the 'www' for a copy of, even if only a single, episode. No damned luck.

'Pretty wild stuff?'. Well, there was this one time. Was in my final year at the university. Had had some 'self-taught' training in Kendo, and Karate. *You'd be surprised how much tv, some reading material, endless motivation, and a sparring partner, can do for 'yer'*. Went so far as to have a local blacksmith (reluctantly) forge me a makeshift Japanese Katana, complete with a 'Tsuba' - that square or oval metal part that separates the blade from the handle. All I had to do was wrap cheap fabric and some foamy material around the handle, and seal with 'duck-like' tape and voila: an amateur-made Japanese Katana was born. Did plenty sparring with that one. Even tried the blindfolded stunt above (remember?) with it and my, rather brave, volunteer came off unscathed (mostly because the watermelon only slit a third of the way through).

So, this day on school campus, I had this capricious drive to pick up that makeshift Katana I had made, stuff it in a tennis racket bag (took some tucking in), walk the mile or so distance from hostel to the popular 'lagoon front' lining  the northern edge of the campus, and set about some whimsical training session that was both foolhardy and blissful.

Turned out some fraternity rites were scheduled at precisely the same time, and general location. So, there I was, doing Karate moves I was never taught by any sensei, with fake Katana strung at my back (Ninja fashion), feeling all 'space samurai' (or maybe ninja) in that deserted part of the campus grounds that time of night.

'You're going to get a serious pounding', came next from somewhere in the dark within maybe a 5-meter radius. Unfazed, I simply tried to determine where that meaningless (well, I was invincible...I believed) threat came from. A burly guy walks up within striking distance with nothing in the way of disguise and stares down at me (I *am* only 5'8). He said nothing else, and the next (very) few seconds saw him flanked by maybe half a dozen 'minions' staring similarly condescendingly at me. It was dark, but I could see the threat well enough. Funny thing was, I welcomed it. I *was* really looking for some live action at the time to justify the intense, and sometimes rather grueling, training sessions I put myself through. To skip the rather tempting histrionics, I saw the light of day with nay a bruise or any manifest scaring I typically *should* have come off with (at least) from that encounter. How?

Fought off a couple guys with self-taught Karate moves that panned out mysteriously, for starters. Guy with the initial threat stayed practically motionless the whole time. First wave of minions dispatched. Silence. Head honcho smiles, then advances toward me. Intent was clear: he was going to bring the hurt. Still unfazed, I unswung my 'trusty' (but really trustless) Katana, slowly (like in the movies) unsheathed only about a quarter of its full length, but enough so the diminishing moonlight could reflect weak but theatrically effective light off the blade. Stopped dead in his advance he did; looked at the blade, then me, then back at the blade, and silently stepped back into the shadows, minions and all. Triumph! You know, he said the, 'you're going to get a pounding' part like that mob guy in one of the 'Johnny Bravo' episodes who threatened Johnny, 'I'm gonna gut you like a kipper'. No idle threat, if you consider Johnny's reaction. I was high on some euphoric sense of combat capability from dubiously acquired martial arts skills; and even as I didn't have any formal training, I could successfully deflect an imminent threat to my 'stable' wellbeing. Don't ever, ever, ever underestimate the power of your mind to push you through perceived limitations. It could all easily have gone south and I'd be having someone I probably never even met give some unearned eulogy afterward. But I gave off an aura of strength and combat skill that made the required, life-saving impression.

I was euphoric, as I mentioned, and obviously didn't fully grasp the danger. But I had a mindset, hard as diamond, that I could hold my own. It radiated all the way to the deadly opponent and, I stayed in one piece. Now, if all that seemed a tad too theatrical to be factual, I offer this: some of the best stories really do shoot from real-life experiences.

Must have told that little story to half a dozen or so people in my life and I'm pretty sure none of them took me seriously - the missy, my number-one doubter. Sometimes I wonder myself. The threat to my life and precious limbs was no joke though; my response, absolutely foolhardy. I was damned lucky to have my hide intact to this day to tell the story one more time.

Had (reasonable) cause to use those self-taught martial arts skills (but never again the fake katana) a few times more after that episode. However, not even in my best (or worst) 'fool-yourself day' did I ever, ever wish for another encounter as mortally dramatic as that one.

So, unless you have a priceless warrior Katana made from metal alloy that can cut most things (they do have them), kick-ass karate moves you genuinely learned at a bona fide dojo, and actual Master Kendo skills, you really, really want to beat it in a situation like my lagoon-front brush. No fun and games I assure you.

What did all that have to do with my journey?

Would probably have ended this all with no need for a 'part two'. Except that, that dramatic episode above came directly back at me in a most unexpected manner. A manner that has everything to do with my journey going in exciting new directions. 'Expect the unexpected' (Terrahawk's Dr. Ninestein). If you know, you know.

December 22<sup>nd</sup>, 2020.

Went out to get some takeaway pizza from a local joint and, right there, directly ahead of me in the line that formed, was my 'would-be assailant' in the episode above. He looked back a couple seconds to regard a family member asking a question from the sidelines. And, that's when I caught that face. Twenty-one years ago it was I saw it last. And in half light! Episode came rushing in like backed-up water in a hose let loose in a container. A few minutes later, I walked up and said these words, "you're going to get a pounding". A lot happened in the following few days far too 'juicy' to let pass.

So, the unexpected new turn? Still living it. I got no idea where it's all headed, but I *will* tell it all.

One thing is clear, so far: My journey – fitness after forty – is nowhere near its end.

# *About the Author*

*Ethan Grove*

Not a whole lot here. Really. Not.

Except, perhaps, that I actually am human. And yes, I do have a degree in Exercise Physiology obtained from a fairly reputable university here on planet earth, so I just might know a little something about the subject matter.

I chose to be cryptic in this section because I have a clear and present phobia for profiling. I think there's too much of it in this our dear world.

One's work should be judged on the basis of 'the work', and pretty much nothing else.

In the end, I'm just the guy next door who needed to share what he deemed a worthwhile story that hopefully touches.